The Tension Headache Pain Relief Guide

Home Remedies to Eliminate Pain Due to Tension Headaches

Table of Contents

Introduction

I want to thank you and congratulate you for downloading the book, "The Tension Headache Pain Relief Guide: Home Remedies to Eliminate Pain Due to Tension Headaches."

This book contains proven steps and strategies on how to get rid of the pain associated with tension headaches through easy home remedies.

Tension headaches, while not entirely debilitating, are often nuisances. Life would be so much better without them. When dealing with headache pain, it is important to know your options. Sure, there are plenty of OTC medications for combating tension headaches. There's Tylenol, Motrin, Aleve, and much much more. The problem with these quick fixes is the unwanted side effects that accompanies most of them. Why not opt for safer, more natural ways to fight those pesky tension headaches?

Within the pages of this book are various home remedies you can try the next time a tension headache attacks. The best thing about the remedies in this book is that they are all-natural, and therefore they are safe and virtually free of adverse side effects. So skip the NSAIDs, and let nature treat your tension headache instead!

Thanks again for downloading this book, I hope you enjoy it!

Chapter 1:
Understanding the Different Types of Headaches

Before we delve into the world of tension headaches, it is helpful to know and understand the different types of headaches first. Many of us often mistake migraines or sinus headaches with tension headaches, and vice versa. In reality, these headaches are very different. Being able to distinguish between the various types of headaches will enable you to recognize and properly treat tension headaches.

Sinus Headache: When an infection strikes, your sinuses may become inflamed, thus causing a headache that is often accompanied by fever. Headaches caused by a sinus infection are readily treated through the use of antibiotics.

Cluster Headache: A cluster headache is a severe type of headache that occurs in cycles or groups. It is a headache that occurs suddenly, and the pain associated with it is often debilitating and limited to one side of the head. Typically, watery eyes and a runny nose accompany a cluster headache. Cluster headaches tend to affect more men than women.

Migraine Headache: A migraine is a recurrent headache that typically affects one side of the head. It is characterized by a painful, throbbing sensation, and is often accompanied by nausea, sensitivity to light or sound, and disturbed vision. The pain associated with migraine headaches is often severe and so debilitating that it can actually interfere with your daily activities. Migraines can last anywhere from several hours to several days. They can begin in childhood, adolescence, or adulthood.

Rebound Headache: Ironically, long-term overuse of medicines used to treat headaches can cause rebound headaches. This is because taking too much pain medications can trigger the brain to become overexcited, thus causing more headaches. Rebound headaches will cease to occur when you begin refraining from taking painkillers.

Tension Headache: Often called "stress headaches," tension headaches are the most common type of headaches among adults. This type of headache is characterized by a constant pressure at the temples, around the neck or forehead, or the back of the head. The degree of pain associated with a tension headache varies, with some describing the ache as mild while others describe it as moderate to severe. A tension headache can last anywhere from half an hour to several days. It often occurs during the day when physical and mental activities are at their peak.

There are two categories of tension headaches: chronic and episodic. Episodic tension headaches happen less than 15 days in a month. They have the potential to become chronic. Chronic tension headaches, on the other hand, occur more than 15 days a month. In some cases, chronic tension headaches attack on a daily basis or are continuous.

Chapter 2:
Symptoms and Causes

Symptoms

The following symptoms may be mild or severe:

- A tightness around your forehead that feels like a rubber band

- An ache at your temples, the back of your neck or head, or your forehead

- Tender scalp or tender muscles in your neck and shoulders

Causes

The exact cause of tension headaches is difficult to pinpoint. However, experts believe that increased sensitivity to stress and muscle tension are responsible. Environmental factors appear to play a role as well.

Possible Triggers

- Stress: It is the leading trigger of tension headaches. Stress may be mental or emotional.

- Inadequate rest

- Sleep deprivation

- Hunger

- Overexertion

- Poor posture

- Anxiety

- Being overweight

- Deadlines at work or school

- Starting or losing a job

- Having a new child

- Buying a new house

- Preparing for exams

- Having a difficult family life

Conventional Treatments

The goal of conventional treatments for tension headaches is to relieve current pain and to prevent future headache occurrences. Preventive action involves taking medications such as antidepressants, muscle relaxants, and painkillers. Avoiding the triggers of tension headaches is also a way to prevent further attacks.

Remember: Medications don't cure headaches, but rather, they provide you with temporary relief. Over-the-counter painkillers tend to lose their effectiveness over time. Furthermore, all medications come with side effects. Worse, medications such as antidepressants and muscle relaxants have the potential for dependence. For these reasons, more and more people are turning to alternative medicines and treatments. You shouldn't rely too heavily on prescription and OTC medications when dealing with tension headaches. Consider giving natural treatments a try—or at least, the benefit of the doubt.

Chapter 3:
Aromatherapy for Tension Headaches

Aromatherapy is a form of all-natural healing that uses essential oils and other aromatics for treating a variety of diseases and ailments. It was developed in ancient China, and is still widely used in modern times. When practiced correctly, aromatherapy can be effective at combating tension headaches.

Since stress is the most common cause of tension headaches, we will mostly be looking into the essential oils that are known for their stress-busting properties.

Lavender Essential Oil: Here is one natural solution for treating tension headaches. Not only does lavender smell wonderful, it also possesses soothing qualities that promote stress-relief and relaxation. The anti-inflammatory effects of lavender essential oil also makes it an effective treatment for tension headaches as it helps in dilating blood vessels.

Lavender essential oil is relatively gentle in comparison with other oils. Thus, it is safe to apply lavender oil topically without diluting it.

For a quick tension headache fix, add 2 drops of lavender oil to 2 cups of water, then inhale the steam.

Basil Essential Oil: Basil oil has been used for centuries in treating headaches and migraines. Because basil acts as a powerful muscle relaxant, basil essential oil is highly effective at treating headaches caused by muscle tension. Basil essential oil works best when combined with lavender essential oil, as their properties complement each other.

To use basil essential oil for tension headaches, dilute it with a carrier oil first, such as almond or coconut oil. Then, massage a drop or two of the essential and carrier oil mixture into your temples, forehead, or the back of your neck.

Peppermint Essential Oil: Those who suffer from tension headaches can benefit greatly from the therapeutic power of peppermint essential oil. It has both vaso-dilating and vaso-constricting properties, which promote proper blood flow. Tension headaches can sometimes result from poor blood flow. Thus, inhaling peppermint essential oil can treat tension headaches by opening and closing the blood vessels in your body.

For an on-the-go tension headache remedy, simply put several drops of peppermint essential oil in a tinted glass vial. Whenever a tension headache attacks, open the vial and wave it under your nose. This remedy is perfect for anyone who suffers from tension headaches at work during midday.

Eucalyptus Essential Oil: Eucalyptus is a rich source of cineole. Cineole is said to be a powerful anti-inflammatory and expectorant. Not only does eucalyptus essential oil open up air passages, it also alleviates headache pain. Use eucalyptus essential oil for treating tension headaches like you would peppermint essential oil.

Rosemary Essential Oil: Rosemary is yet another oil used in aromatherapy for treating all types of headaches. In terms of tension headaches, rosemary essential oil alleviates muscle tension when it is applied directly on problem areas. Relieving muscle tension in the head, neck, or shoulders is one way to remedy tension headaches. Basil essential oil also reduces stress and anxiety.

To use rosemary essential oil for treating tension headaches, simply incorporate 10 drops into a warm bath. Soak for at least 30 minutes while self-massaging.

Frankincense Essential Oil: This essential oil has been used to alleviate headache pain in the past. Frankincense even has the potential to prevent the onset of tension headaches. Frankincense essential oil soothes away the pounding pain associated with chronic tension headaches.

During a tension headache occurrence, try rubbing a drop of frankincense essential oil onto the roof of your mouth. If you can't tolerate the taste of the oil, massage 2 drops into your temples and forehead instead.

Patchouli Essential Oil: This essential oil is most commonly used in aromatherapy for stress relief. It promotes nerve relaxation and cleanses the mind Patchouli essential oil possesses antidepressant properties which make it effective at suppressing volatile emotions and keeping anxiety under control. When used regularly, patchouli oil will keep you rooted in a state of calm.

To use patchouli essential oil in the treatment of tension headaches, simply add several drops into your diffuser. Lay down in a cool, dim place and inhale the aroma.

Marjoram Essential Oil: In ancient times, the Greeks used marjoram for therapeutic purposes. They prepared marjoram oils to use as a relaxant and to calm muscle spasms. Perhaps marjoram's most notable property is analgesic. Marjoram essential oil is extremely effective in treating muscle tension and the pain associated with tension-type headaches.

To use marjoram essential oil for easing muscle tension, massage a small amount of the oil into the tense areas of your body. You can even add 2 drops to a hot or cold compress and apply the compress onto problem areas such as your scalp. For headache relief, simply dilute 2 or 3 drops of marjoram essential oil with an ounce of a carrier oil of your choice. Massage the oil into your temples, neck, or forehead.

Helichrysum Essential Oil: Helichrysum is especially helpful for muscle tension that results in a tension headache. The oil is known for its restorative, anti-inflammatory, and analgesic properties—all of which are helpful in treating tension headaches.

To use helichrysum essential oil for treating tension headaches, try adding a dozen drops to a hot bath. Incorporating 2 cups of Epsom salt into your bathwater will enhance the effect of the helichrysum bath soak.

Roman Chamomile Essential Oil: Roman chamomile offers users its sedative and anti-inflammatory properties. It is useful for nighttime tension headache routines.

Try making a cotton or tissue diffuser by adding 1-2 drops of roman chamomile essential oil to a cotton ball or tissue. Place the diffuser into your pillowcase and sleep with it at night.

Rose Essential Oil: Rose oil is perfect for those who suffer from stress-induced tension headaches. It provides relief from stress, anxiety, and depression. If you want to treat tension headaches in style, then rose essential oil is the oil for you. (Rose essential oil is one of the most expensive oils on the market.) Since rose essential oil is so potent, a miniscule amount is all it takes to get the job done.

Use rose essential oil in a warm bath or in a cotton diffuser to relieve tension headaches.

Vanilla Essential Oil: It is believed that the soothing properties of vanilla essential oil stems from its scent's resemblance to breast milk. Vanilla oil has the ability to clear the mind and induce a state of calm. In this regard, vanilla oil is an effective stress-buster. The analgesic properties of vanilla essential oil make it beneficial for tension headaches.

To use vanilla essential oil for tension headache relief, add a drop to a glass of water, and drink away. Doing so will significantly dull tension headaches.

Bergamot Essential Oil: Bergamot oil is widely used in alternative medicine to cure depression, anxiety, and headaches. It has a sweet, fruity aroma that is said to be both uplifting and relaxing. In cases of tension headaches, bergamot essential oil serves as a potent analgesic by eliminating pain and triggering the release of certain hormones that block pain signals.

To use bergamot essential oil, you can make an aromatic bath by adding 10-12 drops into your bathwater. Soaking in bergamot and inhaling its citrusy aroma will go a long way in relieving stress and muscle tension. You can also use bergamot essential oil as a daily supplement. Consider adding 1-2 drops of bergamot oil to a glass of water or orange juice, and drink every morning.

Sandalwood Essential Oil: Sandalwood is helpful for treating tension headaches, especially if your headache is related to stress. To use sandalwood essential oil in aromatherapy, add 2-3 drops to a bowl of boiling water and inhale the vapors the next time a tension headache attacks.

Ginger Essential Oil: The oil extracted from gingerroot is used in both traditional and alternative medicine. As a natural analgesic and anti-inflammatory, ginger essential oil is extremely effective for treating pain related to tension headaches, stiff muscles, and migraines. Ginger essential oil is also a stress-buster as it possesses stimulating qualities.

You can add 10 drops of ginger oil to a warm bath, 1 drop on a cotton ball, or 2 drops on a handkerchief. For a stress- and pain-relieving massage oil, add 2-3 drops of ginger essential oil to an ounce of extra virgin olive oil and apply topically to the forehead and other problem areas.

Chapter 4:
Plant and Herbal Remedies

Natural treatments doesn't stop with essential oils. Nature thrives with many other treatment forms. You don't have to extract oils and distill plants to benefit from them. This chapter lists various herbs and plants that have the capability of alleviating headache pain and treating tension headaches.

Feverfew: Feverfew is mostly used in alternative medicine as an herbal headache treatment. Feverfew is available in tablet form or freeze-dried capsules. If tension headaches tend to affect you more often during midday, try popping a feverfew pill after lunch. Alternatively, you can grow your own feverfew at home and prepare the leaves in a soothing herbal tea. Feverfew is safe to use every day. In fact, daily use of feverfew is recommended for optimal effect.

Feverfew should be used with caution during pregnancy or if you are breastfeeding. It is not recommended for use in children younger than 2 years of age.

Flaxseed: Flaxseed is a rich source of omega-3 fatty acids—a substance known for its anti-inflammatory effects. Because of this, flaxseed is excellent for relieving headache pain. Flaxseed must be ground to achieve the best results. Ground flaxseed is readily available in health food stores. Begin curing your tension headache today by incorporating one tablespoon of ground flaxseed into your food and beverages. Flaxseed can be mixed into virtually anything—your morning coffee, a smoothie, cake batter, and soups.

Buckwheat: Buckwheat contains rutin, a potent flavanoid and antioxidant that plays a key role in reducing pain associated with tension headaches. Rutin stimulates the secretion of certain hormones known for blocking pain signals. You can benefit from the therapeutic effects of buckwheat by consuming buckwheat honey—which is available in most health food stores.

Butterbur: Butterbur helps in the treatment of migraines, but recent research shows that the herb has a positive effect on tension headaches as well. Butterbur may decrease both the frequency and intensity of tension headaches. You can boil butterbur roots and inhale the steam, or make an herbal tea with butterbur leaves.

Dandelion: The roots of dandelions contains essential vitamins and nutrients that may help in reducing the dull pain associated with tension headaches. You can prepare a cup of dandelion tea to drink daily or when tension headaches strike. Feel free to use either dandelion root powder or actual dandelion roots that are rinsed clean. To make the therapeutic tea, simply boil together a teaspoon of dandelion, a cup of water, and a piece of cinnamon bark for 5-10 minutes. Strain the tea and sweeten it with a drizzle of honey. Pain relief is as simple as that!

Mint: The two primary components of mint, menthol and menthone, are effective at alleviating headache pain. You can make a paste by crushing mint through the implementation of a mortar and pestle. Spread this paste onto your forehead or the back of your neck. Doing so will provide you with a cooling and pain relieving effect for your tension headache.

Rosemary: Rosemary contains rosmarinic acid, which is a powerful anti-inflammatory. You can prepare a therapeutic herbal tea by boiling a teaspoon each of sage and rosemary in one cup of water. Strain, and drink this tea every night.

For optimal effect, drink this rosemary-sage tea twice a day—upon waking and before bedtime.

Cloves: Like mint, cloves has both cooling and pain-relieving properties, which are both useful for treating tension-related headache pain. Treat cloves like potpourri and crush a handful in a handkerchief before tying the small bundle off. When a tension headache strikes, simply put the sack against your nose and breathe deeply. Cloves is also available in oil form, which may be applied topically to your forehead and temples.

Chapter 5:
Pain Relief through Lifestyle Changes, Good Habits, and Alternative Treatments

Treating tension headaches can be as easy as tweaking your lifestyle habits. You can improve your health and well-being by eliminating bad habits and adopting new ones. Remember, pain medications are not a substitute for dealing with the stressors and triggers that may be causing your tension headaches.

As you may remember from Chapter 2, tension headaches can result from mundane things like poor posture and diet. Sometimes it's best to target the root of a tension headache in order to effectively treat it. The following lifestyle tips might just be the solution your tension headache needs.

Biofeedback: Biofeedback is a technique that is useful for controlling the various functions of your body. It involves the use of a monitor to measure your brain waves, heart rate, blood pressure, and even the degree of muscle tension. This method of treatment is effective in dealing with tension headaches because it allows you to improve your health by using the signals your own body emits. Biofeedback teaches you to ease muscle tension to treat existing tension headaches and prevent future attacks. By your own efforts, you can, in fact, remedy your tension headache.

Relaxation Exercises: Practicing relaxation exercises is helpful in treating and managing tension headaches as doing so reduces stress by a significant amount. Consider taking up the art of meditation, practice breathing deeply, or do visualization exercises. All of these exercises are easy to do and will go a long way in dealing with your tension headaches.

Self-Massage: You don't have to splurge at a spa for a soothing massage that relieves stress and muscle tension. Massaging your own body works just as well. Reduce the symptoms of an ongoing tension headache by rubbing circles into your temples or squeezing the back of your neck. Give yourself a good head massage while you're in the shower. Perhaps you'd like to use some of the essential oils mentioned in Chapter 3 in your massage routine. If so, feel free to dilute any one of the oils with a carrier oil like jojoba or sweet almond oil, and massage it into your problem areas. You can even mix-and-match the oils to create your own special massage blend.

Change Your Diet: This is one of the most beneficial home remedies for reducing pain associated with tension headaches. Certain foods affect the frequency and intensity of tension headaches. Such foods include MSG, chocolate, caffeinated beverages, meats containing nitrates, and peanut butter. Keeping track of these trigger foods is made possible through the use of a food diary.

DIY Scalp Massage: You can alleviate headache pain by giving yourself a scalp massage. A scalp massage releases forehead and scalp tension. First, find a quiet place, sit down, and get comfortable. The less distractions, the better. Place your fingers on your forehead, with your thumbs on your temples. Apply light pressure, then release. Move your fingers up your forehead, taking your thumbs with them, and repeat the pressure. Keep moving your fingers up slightly until they are resting on the back of your skull. There is an area at the base of your skull that, when massaged, provides relief from tension headache pain. Make sure to massage this area as well. You can also massage reflex points on your hands and feet to reduce headache pain.

Acupuncture: Acupuncture is a form of complementary medicine that entails the insertion of fine needles into key points of the body. The goal of acupuncture is to realign the flow of energy in the body by stimulating these key points in order to alleviate pain and treat a variety of health conditions. Treating tension headaches may call for pricking areas on the forehead, neck, scalp, temples, or shoulders. It has been said that acupuncture provides as much relief as conventional pain medications.

Stretching: Practicing stretch exercises is helpful for tension headaches that result from muscle tension—which contributes greatly to pain. Try doing shoulder shrugs and neck isometrics the next time you sense a tension headache looming. It is recommended to stretch twice a day—in the mornings and evenings—and to repeat each stretch exercise 5 times.

Aerobics: Aerobics is any vigorous exercise such as briskly walking or swimming. It is designed to improve heart and lung health. Doing aerobics regularly will prevent muscle tension and the occurrence of tension headaches. Aerobics can also decrease the intensity of pain during an ongoing attack.

Yoga: Yoga is a Hindu discipline that involves simple meditation, breath control, and the adoption of specific postures to promote health and relaxation. Practicing yoga as a form of headache therapy will significantly reduce the frequency and severity of tension headaches. In some cases, yoga, when paired with other alternative medicines, cured tension headaches altogether.

Hot and Cold Compresses: This form of tension headache therapy is completely risk-free. Neck tightness can be alleviated by applying a hot compress onto the back of the neck. For pulsing tension headaches, apply an ice cube on both temples. Lowering the temperature of the brain lining actually reduces the degree of pain in cases of tension headaches and migraines.

Avoid Nitrates and Nitrites: These substances are known to induce tension headaches, as well as other headache types. They can be found in sweets, junk food, alcohol, and processed meats. Decreasing your intake of these trigger foods—or even better, completely eliminating them from your diet—will prevent the onset of tension headaches.

Gingerroot: Ginger is extremely effective in treating all forms of headaches. You already learned how to use ginger essential oil for treating tension headaches, so here's how to use fresh gingerroot as an alternative medicine:

Begin by peeling off the skin from one thumb-sized piece of ginger. Cut the ginger into thin slices, and throw the pieces into a saucepan. Add 2 cups of water to the saucepan and boil for 15 minutes. Take the ginger water off the heat, and let it cool. You may add a tablespoon of honey to sweeten the mixture if you please. Drink the ginger water to get rid of tension headache pain.

Tea Tree Oil: Tea tree oil is a natural anti-inflammatory. Use it to reduce tension headache pain due to inflammation. To relieve pain, apply tea tree oil onto your forehead, temples, and neck. Rub the oil in until your skin fully absorbs it. Doing so will provide you with much needed pain relief.

Vinegar: Vinegar is multi-purpose, but who knew it could be used to relieve pain due to tension headaches? Vinegar works by protecting brain cells which receive pain signals. Soak a wash cloth in a bowl of vinegar. Then, lay the cloth onto your forehead, scalp, shoulders, or neck—wherever the pain is most concentrated. Leave the cloth on for 30 minutes before taking a cool shower. Alternatively, you can take a hot aromatic shower by adding 3 drops of one of the essential oils listed in Chapter 3 to your shower floor.

Cayenne Pepper: Capsaicin, the active ingredient in cayenne pepper, is a natural painkiller. Eating spicy foods in general will help alleviate tension headache symptoms. During an attack, try incorporating half a teaspoon of ground cayenne pepper or red pepper flakes into your food. Alternatively, you can take cayenne pepper capsules when a tension headache strikes.

Magnesium: Magnesium is beneficial for easing muscle tension. It also keeps your nerves from becoming too excited, thus preventing tension headaches from occurring. 400 grams of magnesium is all your body needs to combat tension headaches. You can take magnesium daily magnesium supplements, or eat foods that are rich in magnesium, such as salmon, flaxseed, quinoa, and pumpkin seeds.

Omega-3 Fatty Acids: These fatty acids serve in the treatment of tension headaches by acting as potent anti-inflammatories. By protecting the cells in your brain and dilating blood vessels, omega-3 fatty acids provide relief from pain. Getting your daily fix of omega-3s is as easy as eating more fish and nuts.

Vitamin B2: Also known as riboflavin, vitamin B2 is considered to be nature's way of getting rid of headaches. Broccoli, lamb, asparagus, and yogurt are all excellent sources of vitamin B2. Increasing your daily intake of vitamin B2 will go a long way in reducing the severity of tension headaches and preventing future occurrences.

Water: Dehydration is known to trigger headaches and worsen the symptoms of an ongoing tension headache. Drinking a tall glass of cool water as soon as the symptoms of tension headaches start will prevent the incidence of severe and prolonged pain.

Acupressure: When pressed, the L14 acupressure point helps in relieving pain due to headaches. The L14 pressure point is located between your thumb and forefinger; it is the fleshy area between these two fingers. Press this area for one minute, then repeat on your hand.

Conclusion

Thank you again for downloading this book!

I hope this book was able to help you to recognize tension headaches and that it provided you with a comprehensive list of home remedies for you to try at home.

The next step is to take what you've learned in this book, and apply it to your daily life. I hope you know how to manage, prevent, treat, and eliminate the pain associated with those pesky tension headaches that come and go. Remember, muscle tension, stress, and unhealthy habits are the leading triggers of tension headaches. Avoiding stressors and triggers could very well be the cure for tension headaches.

Finally, if you enjoyed this book, then I'd like to ask you for a favor, would you be kind enough to leave a review for this book on Amazon? It'd be greatly appreciated!

Thank you and good luck!